Renal Diet Food List Reference For Kidney Disease

Joel Oliver

Copyright © 2024 Joel Oliver

All rights reserved. No part of this publication may be reproduced, distributed, or transmitted in any form or by any means, including photocopying, recording, or other electronic or mechanical methods, without the prior written permission of the publisher, except in the case of brief quotations embodied in critical reviews and certain other noncommercial uses permitted by copyright law.

Disclaimer:

The information in this book is intended for educational and informational purposes only. The author and publisher make no representations or warranties with respect to the accuracy, applicability, or completeness of the content. The information is provided with the understanding that the author and publisher are not rendering medical, legal, or professional advice. Always seek the advice of a qualified professional with any questions you may have regarding a medical condition or any other subject matter.

Table of Contents

INTRODUCTION 5
    UNDERSTANDING KIDNEY DISEASE 5
    IMPORTANCE OF DIET IN MANAGING KIDNEY DISEASE 6
    OVERVIEW OF THE RENAL DIET 6

CHAPTER1 8
BASICS OF THE RENAL DIET 8
    KEY NUTRIENTS TO MONITOR 8
    FLUID MANAGEMENT 9
    SODIUM AND POTASSIUM CONTROL 9
    PROTEIN INTAKE CONSIDERATIONS 10

CHAPTER2 12
FOOD GROUPS AND 12
THEIR IMPACT 12
    FRUITS 12
    VEGETABLES 13
    GRAINS 14
    PROTEINS 15
    DAIRY AND ALTERNATIVES 16

CHAPTER3 17
SAMPLE MEAL PLANS 17
    BREAKFAST IDEAS 17
    LUNCH OPTIONS 18
    DINNER SUGGESTIONS 19
    SNACKS AND DESSERTS 20

CHAPTER4 21
SPECIAL CONSIDERATIONS 21
    MANAGING DIABETES WITH KIDNEY DISEASE 21
    ADJUSTING DIET FOR DIFFERENT STAGES OF KIDNEY DISEASE 22
    TRAVELING AND EATING OUT 23
    SUPPLEMENTS AND THEIR ROLE 24

CHAPTER 5 26
RECIPES 26
BREAKFAST RECIPES 26
LUNCH RECIPES 28
DINNER RECIPES 31
SNACK RECIPES 33
DESSERT RECIPES 35
CONCLUSION 38
RESOURCES AND TOOLS 40
RECOMMENDED COOKBOOKS AND WEBSITES 40
FOOD DIARY TEMPLATES 41
NUTRITIONAL INFORMATION SOURCES 42
GLOSSARY OF TERMS 43
COMMON TERMS IN RENAL DIET 43
NUTRITIONAL TERMS 45
REFERENCES 47

Introduction

Understanding Kidney Disease

Kidney disease, often known as renal disease, comprises a spectrum of disorders that compromise the kidneys' capacity to operate effectively. The kidneys are crucial organs responsible for filtering waste products and excess fluids from the blood, controlling electrolytes, and creating hormones that support different body activities, including blood pressure regulation and red blood cell synthesis.

Chronic Kidney Disease (CKD) is a progressive decrease of kidney function over time, generally caused by underlying diseases such as diabetes, hypertension, or glomerulonephritis. CKD is defined by the steady decline of kidney function, which can eventually lead to End-Stage Renal Disease (ESRD) or renal failure, where the kidneys are no longer able to perform their important duties. **Acute Kidney Injury (AKI)**, on the other hand, is a quick and severe loss in kidney function, often arising from acute sickness or injury.

Understanding renal illness entails recognizing the symptoms and consequences that occur as kidney function declines. Symptoms may include edema, weariness, abnormalities in urine output, and elevated blood pressure. Effective therapy of renal disease involves a diverse strategy, with nutrition playing a significant role in reducing symptoms and decreasing disease development.

Importance of Diet in Managing Kidney Disease

Diet plays a vital role in controlling renal disease by helping to manage the buildup of waste products and excess fluids in the body. An adequate renal diet can help alleviate symptoms, lower the risk of complications, and enhance overall quality of life.

Key dietary goals for managing kidney disease include:

- **Controlling Sodium Intake:** Excessive salt can lead to fluid retention and high blood pressure, which can exacerbate kidney disease. A low-sodium diet helps to regulate blood pressure and minimize fluid buildup.
- **Managing Potassium Levels:** Potassium is a vital mineral that can become high in kidney disease, leading to serious cardiac rhythm abnormalities. A renal diet frequently includes advice to restrict high-potassium foods and monitor potassium levels.
- **Regulating Protein Intake:** While protein is required for overall health, excessive protein can place additional strain on the kidneys. A renal diet typically entails limiting protein consumption to meet nutritional needs while lowering kidney workload.
- **Controlling Phosphorus**: Elevated phosphorus levels can contribute to bone and cardiovascular issues. Foods high in phosphorus are generally avoided in a renal diet to maintain appropriate phosphorus levels.
- **Fluid Management**: Proper fluid intake is vital, especially in patients with severe renal disease. Monitoring and regulating fluid consumption helps to control fluid balance and prevent problems.

A carefully planned renal diet can help control symptoms, reduce the need for drugs, and halt the progression of kidney disease. It also provides an opportunity for patients to take an active role in their health management through dietary choices.

Overview of the Renal Diet

The renal diet is a customized dietary plan meant to improve kidney function and limit the impact of kidney disease on general health. It is tailored to fit the specific needs of individuals with renal disease and varies based on the stage of the disease and other individual health variables.

Core components of the renal diet include:

- **Low Sodium:** Reducing salt intake helps to manage blood pressure and reduce fluid retention. This frequently means avoiding processed foods, canned items, and high-sodium condiments.
- **Controlled Potassium:** Managing potassium levels requires picking low-potassium fruits and vegetables and avoiding high-potassium choices. Proper portion sizes and food processing practices, such as leaching, can assist minimize potassium concentration in foods.
- **Moderate Protein:** Protein demands are regulated to ensure appropriate nutrition while avoiding strain on the kidneys. Sources of high-quality protein that are friendlier on the kidneys, such as lean meats and egg whites, are commonly recommended.
- **Phosphorus Management**: Phosphorus control comprises avoiding foods high in phosphorus and utilizing phosphate binders if advised. Reading food labels and choosing phosphorus-free alternatives are crucial strategies.
- **Fluid Intake**: Fluid recommendations vary based on individual health condition and renal function. Monitoring and regulating fluid intake is vital to prevent dehydration or fluid excess.

The renal diet is not a one-size-fits-all solution but rather a personalized regimen that takes into account the particular demands and preferences of each individual. By adopting a renal diet, individuals with kidney disease can effectively control their illness, enhance their well-being, and improve their quality of life.

This introduction gives a good foundation for understanding kidney illness, the necessity of dietary control, and the concepts of the renal diet.

Chapter 1

Basics of the Renal Diet

Key Nutrients to Monitor

For individuals with renal disease, monitoring certain nutrients is vital to controlling the condition and minimizing consequences. The major nutrients to focus on are sodium, potassium, phosphorus, and protein, each of which plays a significant part in kidney health and overall well-being.

- **Sodium:** Excess sodium can lead to fluid retention and high blood pressure, which can compromise renal function. It is necessary to monitor and limit sodium consumption to assist maintain blood pressure and decrease fluid buildup.
- **Potassium:** Potassium is necessary for heart and muscle function, but excessive amounts can trigger severe heart arrhythmias. Individuals with kidney disease need to check potassium levels and choose diets that are low in potassium to avoid consequences.
- **Phosphorus:** Phosphorus is crucial for bone health, but high levels can contribute to bone and cardiovascular disorders. The kidneys regulate phosphorus levels, thus limiting dietary phosphorus is vital to prevent imbalances.

- **Protein:** While protein is required for maintaining muscle mass and overall health, excessive protein can place additional strain on the kidneys. Balancing protein intake helps to maintain renal workload and prevent additional damage.

Fluid Management

Fluid control is a key component of the renal diet, particularly for patients with severe kidney disease or those receiving dialysis. Proper fluid consumption helps to maintain hydration levels and prevent issues such as fluid excess or dehydration.

- **Assessing Fluid Needs:** Fluid demands vary based on the stage of renal disease, individual health state, and treatment options. It's crucial to follow instructions set by healthcare specialists to determine the optimal fluid consumption.
- **Managing Fluid Intake**: Monitoring daily fluid intake and output helps to manage fluid balance. This may involve tracking all sources of fluid, including beverages and foods with high water content.
- **Adjusting Fluid Intake**: In cases of fluid retention or low kidney function, it may be necessary to reduce fluid consumption. Conversely, some individuals may require more fluid consumption to stay hydrated. Adhering to dietary recommendations and modifying fluid consumption as needed is key.
- **Signs of Fluid Imbalance**: Monitoring for symptoms such as edema, weight gain, shortness of breath, and changes in urine output can assist identify fluid imbalances and suggest improvements in fluid management.

Sodium and Potassium Control

Controlling salt and potassium consumption is crucial for controlling renal illness and preventing complications. Both minerals have a substantial impact on blood pressure, fluid balance, and overall renal function.

- **Sodium Control:**
  - **Limit Processed Foods:** Processed and packaged foods generally contain excessive quantities of salt. Opt for fresh, healthy foods and utilize herbs and spices for flavoring instead of salt.
  - **Read Food Labels:** Pay attention to salt content on food labels and choose low-sodium or sodium-free options whenever possible.
  - **Cooking Methods:** Use cooking methods that decrease sodium, such as baking, grilling, or steaming, rather than frying or using salt-based spices.
- **Potassium Control:**
  - **Choose Low-Potassium Foods:** Incorporate fruits and vegetables that are low in potassium, such as apples, berries, carrots, and green beans. Avoid high-potassium foods including bananas, oranges, potatoes, and tomatoes.
  - **Portion Sizes:** Even low-potassium foods can contribute to potassium intake if consumed in big quantities. Adhere to appropriate portion sizes to maintain potassium levels effectively.
  - **Food Preparation:** Techniques such as soaking and boiling vegetables can help reduce potassium level. For example, cooking potatoes and eliminating the water can lower potassium levels in the final dish.

Protein Intake Considerations

Managing protein consumption is critical for patients with renal disease, as much protein can increase kidney function while insufficient protein can lead to malnutrition and muscle loss.

- **Balanced Protein Intake:** Strive for a balanced approach by ingesting modest amounts of high-quality protein. Focus on foods that are friendlier on the kidneys, such as lean meats, fish, and egg whites.

- **Types of Protein:**
  - **Animal-Based Proteins:** These include poultry, fish, and lean portions of beef or pork. They are called high-quality proteins because they contain all essential amino acids.
  - **Plant-Based Proteins:** Include alternatives such as tofu, tempeh, and lentils, but be aware of phosphorus content and portion amounts.
- **Timing and Distribution:** Distributing protein consumption evenly throughout the day can assist optimize renal function and minimize excessive strain. Avoid huge quantities of protein in a single meal.
- **Protein Supplements:** In some circumstances, protein supplements may be prescribed to provide nutritional demands without overloading the kidneys. Consult with a healthcare expert before adding supplements to your diet.

By focusing on four critical features of the renal diet, individuals with kidney disease can better control their condition and maintain maximum health. Adhering to dietary standards and working closely with healthcare specialists ensures that nutritional intake is balanced and adapted to individual needs.

This section provides a complete discussion of the fundamental features of the renal diet, addressing the monitoring of important nutrients, fluid management, and the control of sodium, potassium, and protein intake.

Chapter 2
Food Groups and Their Impact

Fruits

Fruits can be a significant element of a renal diet, but it's important to choose kinds that fit within the dietary restrictions of kidney illness, particularly concerns potassium levels.

Low-Potassium Options

For those with renal illness, regulating potassium intake is critical. Here are some low-potassium fruit options:

- **Apples:** A versatile fruit that can be eaten raw, cooked, or baked.
- **Berries:** Blueberries, strawberries, and raspberries are often lower in potassium and strong in antioxidants.
- **Grapes:** Both red and green grapes are lower in potassium compared to other fruits.

- **Peaches:** Fresh or canned peaches (without added sugar) are a fine alternative.
- **Pineapple:** Fresh pineapple delivers a tropical flavor with decreased potassium content.

It's vital to speak with a healthcare expert to establish which fruits are appropriate based on individual potassium levels.

Portion Sizes

Even low-potassium fruits need to be consumed in suitable portion proportions to maintain balanced potassium intake. Standard serving sizes are:

- **Apples:** One medium apple (approximately 3 inches in diameter).
- **Berries:** One cup of fresh berries.
- **Grapes:** One cup of grapes.
- **Peaches:** One medium peach.
- **Pineapple:** One cup of fresh pineapple chunks.

Monitoring portion sizes helps regulate overall potassium consumption while still enjoying a variety of fruits.

Vegetables

Vegetables are an integral element of a healthy diet but must be chosen and prepared carefully in a renal diet to control potassium and salt consumption.

Low-Potassium and Low-Sodium Choices

Select vegetables that are both low in potassium and sodium:

- **Cucumbers:** Low in potassium and salt, perfect for salads and snacking.
- **Bell Peppers:** Red, green, and yellow bell peppers are low in potassium.
- **Cauliflower:** Can be used in numerous meals and has a low potassium content.

- **Green Beans:** Fresh or frozen green beans are low in potassium.
- **Lettuce:** Various forms of lettuce are low in potassium and salt.

Cooking Methods

The manner vegetables are prepared can alter their nutritious content, particularly potassium levels:

- **Boiling:** Boiling veggies and discarding the water might reduce potassium concentration. This procedure is useful for potatoes, carrots, and other root vegetables.
- **Steaming:** Steaming helps maintain most nutrients while lowering potassium compared to boiling.
- **Baking and Roasting:** These procedures can enhance flavor without dramatically reducing potassium levels. Use herbs and spices for enhanced taste.

Grains

Grains give important carbs and energy but should be picked carefully to correspond with a renal diet.

Gluten-Free Options

For persons with renal illness and gluten intolerance, gluten-free grains are necessary:

- **Quinoa:** A full protein and gluten-free grain that is suitable for numerous meals.
- **Rice:** Both white and brown rice are gluten-free, while brown rice has more phosphorus.
- **Buckwheat:** Despite its name, buckwheat is gluten-free and provides a healthy source of protein and fiber.
- **Millet:** A gluten-free grain that can be used as a side dish or in baking.

Whole vs. Refined Grains

- **Whole Grains:** Generally contain more minerals and fiber compared to refined grains, but also more phosphorus. Examples include quinoa and brown rice.
- **Refined Grains:** Lower in phosphorus and potassium but less nutritious. Examples include white rice and refined white bread.

Balancing whole and refined grains while considering phosphorus and potassium content is crucial.

Proteins

Proteins are crucial for sustaining muscle mass and overall health but must be controlled carefully in a renal diet.

Animal Proteins

Animal proteins are high-quality sources of protein but should be consumed in moderation:

- **Chicken:** Lean pieces like breast meat are lower in phosphorus and potassium.
- **Fish:** Varieties such as salmon and tilapia are healthy protein sources but should be monitored for phosphorus content.
- **Egg Whites:** A superb protein source with low phosphorus and potassium.

Plant-Based Proteins

Plant-based proteins can be incorporated in a renal diet but must be chosen wisely:

- **Tofu:** Provides a rich amount of protein and can be utilized in numerous ways.
- **Tempeh:** Fermented soy food with increased protein content, yet it has a modest phosphorus level.
- **Legumes:** Beans and lentils are strong in protein but also phosphorus, so portion control is crucial.

Dairy and Alternatives

Dairy products are a substantial source of calcium and protein but can be heavy in phosphorus and potassium.

Low-Phosphorus Choices

For individuals needing to manage phosphorus levels:

- **Almond Milk:** Often lower in phosphorus compared to cow's milk and can be supplemented with calcium.
- **Rice Milk:** A lower-phosphorus alternative to dairy milk.
- **Coconut Milk:** Can be used as a dairy alternative and is often lower in phosphorus.

Lactose-Free Options

For those with lactose intolerance or sensitivity:

- **Lactose-Free Milk:** Available in numerous forms, including cow's milk and plant-based alternatives.
- **Lactose-Free Yogurt:** Can give beneficial probiotics without the lactose content.
- **Cheese Alternatives:** Look for lactose-free or reduced-lactose choices.

Choosing the correct dairy or dairy replacements helps balance phosphorus and calcium consumption while accommodating dietary needs.

This section offers a thorough discussion of how different food groups effect a renal diet, including practical recommendations for managing nutrient intake and achieving a balanced diet.

Chapter 3

Sample Meal Plans

Breakfast Ideas

Berry Oatmeal

Ingredients:

- 1/2 cup rolled oats
- 1 cup water
- 1/2 cup fresh blueberries
- 1/2 cup fresh strawberries, sliced
- 1 tablespoon honey (optional)
- 1/4 teaspoon cinnamon

Procedure:

1. In a small pot, bring the water to a boil.
2. Add the rolled oats and decrease heat to a simmer.
3. Cook the oats for about 5 minutes, stirring regularly.
4. Stir in the blueberries and strawberries.
5. Cook for an additional 2-3 minutes until the oats are mushy and the fruit is cooked through.
6. Remove from heat and toss in honey and cinnamon if preferred.

Time Frame:

- Preparation Time: 10 minutes
- Yield: 1 serving

Nutritional Value: (Approximate)

- Calories: 300
- Protein: 6g
- Potassium: 250mg
- Phosphorus: 150mg

Alternative Ingredients:

- Substitute honey with maple syrup if preferred.

Lunch Options

Chicken and Vegetable Stir-Fry

Ingredients:

- 1 cup diced chicken breast
- 1 tablespoon olive oil
- 1 cup chopped bell peppers (red, green, yellow)
- 1 cup chopped broccoli
- 1/2 cup sliced carrots
- 2 tablespoons low-sodium soy sauce
- 1 tablespoon cornstarch mixed with 2 tablespoons water

Procedure:

1. Heat the olive oil in a big pan over medium heat.
2. Add the diced chicken and sauté until browned and cooked through, about 5-7 minutes.
3. Add the bell peppers, broccoli, and carrots. Stir-fry for 5 minutes until vegetables are tender-crisp.
4. Stir in the low-sodium soy sauce.
5. Mix the cornstarch with water and add to the pan, stirring until the sauce thickens.
6. Serve hot.

Time Frame:

- Preparation Time: 15 minutes
- Yield: 2 servings

Nutritional Value: (Approximate)

- Calories: 350 per serving
- Protein: 30g
- Potassium: 450mg
- Phosphorus: 200mg

Alternative Ingredients:

- Substitute chicken with tofu for a plant-based option.

Dinner Suggestions

Quinoa and Cauliflower Pilaf

Ingredients:

- 1 cup quinoa
- 2 cups low-sodium vegetable broth
- 1 cup chopped cauliflower
- 1/2 cup diced bell peppers
- 1 tablespoon olive oil
- 1/2 teaspoon turmeric
- Salt and pepper to taste

Procedure:

1. Rinse the quinoa under cool water.
2. In a medium pot, bring the vegetable broth to a boil.
3. Add the quinoa, decrease heat to low, and simmer for 15 minutes.
4. In a large skillet, heat the olive oil over medium heat.
5. Add the cauliflower and bell peppers, simmering until soft, about 5-7 minutes.
6. Stir in the cooked quinoa and turmeric. Season with salt and pepper.
7. Serve warm.

Time Frame:

- Preparation Time: 20 minutes
- Yield: 2 servings

Nutritional Value: (Approximate)

- Calories: 280 per serving
- Protein: 9g
- Potassium: 400mg
- Phosphorus: 160mg

Alternative Ingredients:

- Substitute cauliflower with zucchini or green beans if preferred.

Snacks and Desserts

Apple and Cinnamon Rice Cake

Ingredients:

- 1 rice cake
- 1/2 apple, thinly sliced
- 1/2 teaspoon ground cinnamon
- 1 tablespoon almond butter

Procedure:

1. Spread almond butter evenly over the rice cake.
2. Arrange the apple slices on top of the almond butter.
3. Sprinkle with ground cinnamon.
4. Enjoy as a light and healthful snack.

Time Frame:

- Preparation Time: 5 minutes
- Yield: 1 serving

Nutritional Value: (Approximate)

- Calories: 150
- Protein: 4g
- Potassium: 150mg
- Phosphorus: 70mg

Alternative Ingredients:

- Substitute almond butter with sunflower seed butter if nut-free.

These meal plans and recipes are meant to be nutritious and practical for those on a renal diet, guaranteeing balanced intake of important nutrients while adhering to dietary limitations.

Chapter 4
Special Considerations

Managing Diabetes with Kidney Disease

Managing diabetes and renal illness needs careful coordination of dietary and pharmacological measures to reduce blood sugar levels while sustaining kidney function.

Key Strategies:

- **Monitor Carbohydrate Intake:** Focus on controlling carbohydrate intake to manage blood glucose levels. Choose low-glycemic index foods that have a slower influence on blood sugar, such as whole grains, non-starchy veggies, and legumes.
- **Regular Blood Sugar Monitoring:** Frequent monitoring of blood glucose levels helps to alter insulin or prescription dosages and dietary choices. Aim for constant blood sugar management to prevent problems.
- **Balanced Meals:** Incorporate balanced meals that include lean proteins, healthy fats, and fiber-rich carbohydrates to stabilize blood sugar levels. Avoid excessive sugar and refined carbs, which can contribute to rises in blood glucose.

- **Portion management:** Practice portion management to manage caloric intake and prevent overeating. Small, frequent meals may help in balancing blood sugar levels throughout the day.
- **Consult Healthcare Providers:** Regular visits with a healthcare physician or nutritionist specialized in diabetes and renal disease are crucial. They can provide individualized guidance and changes based on individual health state and treatment goals.

Adjusting Diet for Different Stages of Kidney Disease

The dietary needs and restrictions vary depending on the stage of kidney disease, from early-stage CKD to end-stage renal disease (ESRD).

Early-Stage CKD:

- **Moderate Protein:** Limit protein consumption to avoid renal workload. Include high-quality protein sources and prevent excessive consumption.
- **Balanced Electrolytes:** Monitor potassium and phosphorus levels, making modifications depending on lab results and dietary recommendations.
- **Fluid Management:** Generally less restricted, but individual needs may differ.

Mid-Stage CKD:

- **Strict Sodium and Potassium Control:** Limit sodium and potassium intake more strictly to manage symptoms and avoid further development.
- **Phosphorus Control:** Avoid high-phosphorus diets and consider phosphate binders if prescribed by a healthcare provider.
- **Protein Restriction:** Further restrict protein consumption while ensuring enough nourishment.

End-Stage Renal Disease (ESRD):

- **Dialysis Diet:** If undergoing dialysis, follow particular dietary instructions to control potassium, phosphorus, and fluid balance. This may include very minimal potassium and phosphorus consumption and careful hydration management.
- **Increased Protein Needs:** Dialysis patients often require increased protein intake to compensate for protein loss during dialysis sessions.
- **Specialized Diet:** Adhere to a diet plan tailored to dialysis demands, including limitations on specific nutrients and potential usage of supplements.

Traveling and Eating Out

Traveling and eating out might bring complications for persons with renal illness. Planning and preparation are crucial to maintaining a renal-friendly diet while away from home.

Travel Tips:

- **Plan Ahead:** Research and arrange meals before traveling. Identify restaurants or food options that offer adequate choices and have a plan for how to manage dining out.
- **Pack Snacks:** Carry renal-friendly snacks and meals to avoid relying on limited options while traveling.
- **Communicate Dietary Needs:** When dining out, carefully convey dietary limitations and preferences to restaurant staff. Request adjustments to dishes to match dietary restrictions.
- **Stay Hydrated:** Maintain sufficient hydration, but be careful of fluid limits if applicable. Carry a water bottle and provide access to clean drinking water.

Eating Out Tips:

- **Choose Low-Sodium Options:** Opt for items that are steamed, grilled, or baked rather than fried, and request sauces and dressings on the side.
- **Monitor Portion Sizes:** Be wary with portion sizes and avoid excessive servings of high-potassium or high-phosphorus foods.
- **Ask for Ingredient Information:** Request extensive information on ingredients and preparation processes to make informed choices.

Supplements and Their Role

Supplements can play a supporting role in controlling kidney illness, but they should be used cautiously and under professional advice.

Common Supplements:

- **Vitamin D:** May be advised if there is a deficiency, as kidney disease might impair vitamin D metabolism.
- **Iron:** Often recommended to address anemia associated with chronic renal disease, especially in persons on dialysis.
- **Omega-3 Fatty Acids:** Can provide anti-inflammatory properties and enhance heart health. Consult with a healthcare provider to ensure optimum dosage and suitability.
- **Phosphate Binders:** Used to manage phosphorus levels in the blood, particularly for persons with ESRD.

Precautions:

- **Consult Healthcare Providers:** Always speak with a healthcare provider before starting any new supplements. Some supplements may interact with drugs or impact renal function.
- **Avoid Overuse:** Be cautious of overusing supplements or taking them in excess, since this can lead to imbalances and potential health risks.

- **Choose High-Quality Supplements:** Opt for high-quality, reputable products to assure purity and efficacy.

By addressing these special factors, individuals with kidney illness can better manage their condition and maintain overall health. Each aspect—whether managing diabetes, modifying food according to disease stage, traveling, or using supplements—requires strategic planning and professional advice to obtain optimal outcomes.

This section addresses critical concerns for managing renal illness, focusing on diabetes management, dietary modifications, travel suggestions, and the significance of supplements.

Chapter 5 Recipes

Breakfast Recipes

Spinach and Egg White Muffins

Ingredients:

- 1 cup fresh spinach, chopped
- 6 egg whites
- 1/4 cup diced red bell pepper
- 1/4 cup low-fat milk
- 1/4 teaspoon black pepper
- 1/4 teaspoon garlic powder

Procedure:

1. Preheat the oven to 350°F (175°C) and lightly oil a muffin pan.
2. In a bowl, whisk together egg whites, milk, black pepper, and garlic powder.
3. Stir in chopped spinach and diced bell pepper.
4. Pour the mixture evenly into muffin tin cups.
5. Bake for 20-25 minutes, or until muffins are set and slightly brown on top.
6. Allow to cool before serving.

Time Frame:

- Preparation Time: 10 minutes
- Cooking Time: 25 minutes
- Yield: 6 muffins

Nutritional Value: (Approximate per muffin)

- Calories: 60
- Protein: 6g
- Potassium: 200mg
- Phosphorus: 90mg

Alternative Ingredients:

- Substitute spinach with kale or Swiss chard if preferred.

Chia Seed Pudding with Berries

Ingredients:

- 1/4 cup chia seeds
- 1 cup unsweetened almond milk
- 1 tablespoon maple syrup (optional)
- 1/2 teaspoon vanilla extract
- 1/2 cup mixed berries (blueberries, raspberries)

Procedure:

1. In a dish, blend chia seeds, almond milk, maple syrup, and vanilla essence.
2. Stir thoroughly and let settle for 5 minutes. Stir again to prevent clumping.
3. Cover and chill for at least 2 hours or overnight.
4. Serve topped with mixed berries.

Time Frame:

- Preparation Time: 10 minutes
- Refrigeration Time: 2 hours
- Yield: 1 serving

Nutritional Value: (Approximate)

- Calories: 220
- Protein: 6g
- Potassium: 150mg
- Phosphorus: 120mg

Alternative Ingredients:

- Substitute almond milk with rice milk if preferred.

Overnight Oats with Apples and Cinnamon

Ingredients:

- 1/2 cup rolled oats
- 1/2 cup low-fat milk
- 1/2 apple, diced
- 1/2 teaspoon cinnamon
- 1 tablespoon chopped walnuts (optional)

Procedure:

1. In a jar or container, combine rolled oats, milk, and cinnamon.
2. Stir in diced apple.
3. Cover and refrigerate overnight.
4. Top with walnuts before serving if preferred.

Time Frame:

- Preparation Time: 5 minutes
- Refrigeration Time: Overnight
- Yield: 1 serving

Nutritional Value: (Approximate)

- Calories: 270
- Protein: 8g
- Potassium: 300mg
- Phosphorus: 180mg

Alternative Ingredients:

- Substitute walnuts with almonds or omit if preferred.

Lunch Recipes

Turkey and Cucumber Wrap

Ingredients:

- 1 whole wheat tortilla
- 3 oz. sliced turkey breast (low sodium)
- 1/2 cucumber, sliced thinly
- 1/4 cup shredded lettuce
- 1 tablespoon hummus

Procedure:

1. Spread the hummus evenly over the tortilla.
2. Layer the turkey slices, cucumber, and shredded lettuce on top.
3. Roll the tortilla tightly and slice in half.

4. Serve immediately or wrap in foil for a portable lunch.

Time Frame:

- Preparation Time: 5 minutes
- Yield: 1 wrap

Nutritional Value: (Approximate)

- Calories: 250
- Protein: 20g
- Potassium: 300mg
- Phosphorus: 150mg

Alternative Ingredients:

- Substitute turkey with chicken breast or tofu for a different protein choice.

Greek Quinoa Salad

Ingredients:

- 1 cup cooked quinoa
- 1/2 cup diced cucumber
- 1/2 cup cherry tomatoes, halved
- 1/4 cup sliced olives (low sodium)
- 1/4 cup crumbled feta cheese (optional)
- 1 tablespoon olive oil
- 1 tablespoon lemon juice
- 1/4 teaspoon dried oregano

Procedure:

1. In a large bowl, combine cooked quinoa, cucumber, cherry tomatoes, and olives.
2. In a small bowl, stir together olive oil, lemon juice, and oregano.
3. Pour the dressing over the salad and toss to combine.
4. Top with crumbled feta cheese if using.

Time Frame:

- Preparation Time: 10 minutes
- Yield: 2 servings

Nutritional Value: (Approximate per serving)

- Calories: 280
- Protein: 8g
- Potassium: 300mg
- Phosphorus: 200mg

Alternative Ingredients:

- Substitute feta cheese with a vegan cheese option if preferred.

Chicken and Avocado Salad

Ingredients:

- 1 cup cooked chicken breast, shredded
- 1/2 avocado, diced
- 1 cup mixed greens
- 1/4 cup cherry tomatoes, halved
- 1 tablespoon olive oil
- 1 tablespoon balsamic vinegar
- Salt and pepper to taste

Procedure:

1. In a bowl, combine chicken, avocado, mixed greens, and cherry tomatoes.
2. In a small bowl, whisk together olive oil and balsamic vinegar.
3. Drizzle the dressing over the salad and toss lightly to mix.
4. Season with salt and pepper to taste.

Time Frame:

- Preparation Time: 10 minutes
- Yield: 2 servings

Nutritional Value: (Approximate per serving)

- Calories: 300
- Protein: 25g
- Potassium: 350mg
- Phosphorus: 250mg

Alternative Ingredients:

- Substitute chicken with tofu for a plant-based option.

Dinner Recipes

Lemon Herb Baked Salmon

Ingredients:

- 2 salmon fillets (6 oz. each)
- 1 lemon, sliced
- 1 tablespoon olive oil
- 1 teaspoon dried dill
- 1 teaspoon dried thyme
- Salt and pepper to taste

Procedure:

1. Preheat the oven to 375°F (190°C).
2. Place salmon fillets on a baking pan lined with parchment paper.
3. Drizzle olive oil over the fillets and season with dill, thyme, salt, and pepper.
4. Place lemon slices on top of the fish.
5. Bake for 15-20 minutes, or until salmon is cooked through and flakes readily with a fork.
6. Serve with a side of steamed vegetables or quinoa.

Time Frame:

- Preparation Time: 10 minutes
- Cooking Time: 20 minutes
- Yield: 2 servings

Nutritional Value: (Approximate per serving)

- Calories: 300
- Protein: 25g
- Potassium: 400mg
- Phosphorus: 250mg

Alternative Ingredients:

- Substitute salmon with another fish like tilapia or cod if preferred.

Stuffed Bell Peppers

Ingredients:

- 4 bell peppers (any color)
- 1 cup cooked brown rice
- 1/2 cup cooked lean ground turkey
- 1/2 cup diced tomatoes
- 1/4 cup chopped onions
- 1/4 cup shredded mozzarella cheese (optional)
- 1 teaspoon Italian seasoning

Procedure:

1. Preheat the oven to 375°F (190°C).
2. Cut the tops off the bell peppers and remove seeds and membranes.
3. In a bowl, add cooked rice, ground turkey, chopped tomatoes, onions, and Italian seasoning.
4. Stuff the peppers with the mixture and place in a roasting dish.
5. Top with shredded mozzarella cheese if using.
6. Bake for 25-30 minutes, or until peppers are tender.

Time Frame:

- Preparation Time: 15 minutes
- Cooking Time: 30 minutes
- Yield: 4 servings

Nutritional Value: (Approximate per serving)

- Calories: 280
- Protein: 20g
- Potassium: 400mg
- Phosphorus: 220mg

Alternative Ingredients:

- Substitute ground turkey with lentils for a vegetarian option.

Baked Cod with Lemon and Dill

Ingredients:

- 2 cod fillets (6 oz. each)
- 1 tablespoon olive oil
- 1 lemon, sliced
- 1 teaspoon dried dill
- 1/4 teaspoon black pepper

Procedure:

1. Preheat the oven to 400°F (200°C).
2. Place fish fillets on a baking pan lined with parchment paper.
3. Drizzle with olive oil and season with dill and black pepper.
4. Place lemon slices on top of the fillets.
5. Bake for 15-20 minutes, or until fish flakes easily with a fork.

Time Frame:

- Preparation Time: 10 minutes
- Cooking Time: 20 minutes
- Yield: 2 servings

Nutritional Value: (Approximate per serving)

- Calories: 200
- Protein: 25g
- Potassium: 350mg
- Phosphorus: 200mg

Alternative Ingredients:

- Substitute cod with another white fish like tilapia or haddock.

Snack Recipes

Carrot Sticks with Hummus

Ingredients:

- 1 cup carrot sticks
- 1/4 cup homemade or store-bought hummus (low sodium)

Procedure:

1. Peel and cut carrots into sticks.
2. Serve with hummus for dipping.
3. Enjoy as a quick, healthy snack.

Time Frame:

- Preparation Time: 5 minutes
- Yield: 1 serving

Nutritional Value: (Approximate)

- Calories: 120
- Protein: 4g
- Potassium: 300mg
- Phosphorus: 70mg

Alternative Ingredients:

- Substitute carrots with celery sticks or cucumber slices.

Cucumber and Hummus Bites

Ingredients:

- 1 cucumber, sliced into rounds
- 1/4 cup low-sodium hummus
- Fresh dill for garnish (optional)

Procedure:

1. Arrange cucumber slices on a platter.
2. Top each slice with a small dollop of hummus.
3. Garnish with fresh dill if preferred.
4. Serve immediately.

Time Frame:

- Preparation Time: 5 minutes
- Yield: 1 serving (can be adjusted)

Nutritional Value: (Approximate)

- Calories: 100
- Protein: 3g
- Potassium: 250mg
- Phosphorus: 50mg

Alternative Ingredients:

- Substitute hummus with Greek yogurt dip if preferred.

Baked Sweet Potato Chips

Ingredients:

- 1 large sweet potato
- 1 tablespoon olive oil
- 1/2 teaspoon paprika
- 1/4 teaspoon garlic powder
- Salt to taste

Procedure:

1. Preheat the oven to 400°F (200°C).
2. Peel and slice the sweet potato into thin rounds.
3. Toss with olive oil, paprika, garlic powder, and salt.
4. Spread in a single layer on a baking sheet.
5. Bake for 20-25 minutes, rotating halfway, until crispy.

Time Frame:

- Preparation Time: 10 minutes
- Cooking Time: 25 minutes
- Yield: 1 serving

Nutritional Value: (Approximate)

- Calories: 180
- Protein: 2g
- Potassium: 450mg
- Phosphorus: 40mg

Alternative Ingredients:

- Substitute paprika with a different seasoning blend if preferred.

Dessert Recipes

Baked Apple with Cinnamon

Ingredients:

- 1 medium apple
- 1 teaspoon ground cinnamon
- 1 tablespoon honey (optional)
- 1/4 cup chopped nuts (optional)

Procedure:

1. Preheat the oven to 350°F (175°C).
2. Core the apple and lay it in a baking dish.
3. Sprinkle with cinnamon and drizzle with honey if using.
4. Bake for 20-25 minutes, or until apple is soft.
5. Sprinkle with chopped nuts if desired before serving.

Time Frame:

- Preparation Time: 5 minutes
- Cooking Time: 25 minutes
- Yield: 1 serving

Nutritional Value: (Approximate)

- Calories: 150
- Protein: 2g
- Potassium: 200mg
- Phosphorus: 50mg

Alternative Ingredients:

- Substitute honey with maple syrup or eliminate for a lower sugar option.

Berry Banana Smoothie

Ingredients:

- 1 banana
- 1/2 cup frozen berries (blueberries or strawberries)
- 1/2 cup unsweetened almond milk
- 1 tablespoon chia seeds (optional)

Procedure:

1. In a blender, combine banana, frozen berries, almond milk, and chia seeds if using.
2. Blend until smooth.
3. Pour into a glass and serve immediately.

Time Frame:

- Preparation Time: 5 minutes
- Yield: 1 serving

Nutritional Value: (Approximate)

- Calories: 180
- Protein: 4g
- Potassium: 400mg
- Phosphorus: 60mg

Alternative Ingredients:

- Substitute almond milk with rice milk if preferred.

Cinnamon Baked Pears

Ingredients:

- 2 pears, halved and cored
- 1 tablespoon honey (optional)
- 1/2 teaspoon ground cinnamon
- 1/4 cup chopped nuts (optional)

Procedure:

1. Preheat the oven to 350°F (175°C).
2. Place pear halves in a baking dish.
3. Drizzle with honey if using and sprinkle with cinnamon.
4. Bake for 20-25 minutes, until pears are soft.
5. Top with chopped nuts before serving if preferred.

Time Frame:

- Preparation Time: 5 minutes
- Cooking Time: 25 minutes
- Yield: 2 servings

Nutritional Value: (Approximate per serving)

- Calories: 160
- Protein: 2g
- Potassium: 220mg
- Phosphorus: 50mg

Alternative Ingredients:

- Substitute honey with maple syrup or omit for a lower sugar option.

These dishes give a range of meal options ideal for a renal diet, concentrating on balanced nutrition and flavor while following to dietary limitations.

Conclusion

Embarking on the journey of treating renal disease with nutrition is both a commitment to health and an act of self-care. The renal diet, albeit sometimes complex, provides a life-changing opportunity to reduce disease progression, maintain energy levels, and minimize complications. By learning how individual nutrients like salt, potassium, phosphorus, and protein impact kidney health, you're empowered to make choices that directly benefit your well-being and general quality of life.

While controlling renal illness can initially feel overwhelming, tiny, conscious changes in dietary habits can provide large, permanent gains. Every meal choice becomes a step toward maintaining your kidney function, minimizing pressure on your body, and encouraging longevity. This guide is designed not only to expose you to kidney-friendly foods but also to help you develop practical skills—meal planning, reading nutrition labels, and making thoughtful choices—that enable you to maintain a balanced, gratifying diet even as your health needs alter.

One of the main issues with the renal diet is the regular monitoring of nutritional levels and portion sizes. However, using resources like personalized recipes, dietary lists, and meal-planning templates, this book seeks to simplify the process, making kidney care easy and achievable. As you adapt these practices, you'll find that many kidney-friendly foods are nutritious, enjoyable, and supportive of an overall balanced lifestyle. From full breakfasts to delicious dinners and even occasional treats, you may enjoy a variety of meals without feeling constrained.

As you continue on your path, it's important to realize that each individual's experience with kidney disease is unique. Kidney function and nutritional demands can change over time, and remaining aware and proactive about these variations is crucial. Regularly engaging with healthcare professionals, such as renal dietitians, can assist customize your diet to your unique needs, ensuring that your food choices fit with your current health goals. They can provide tailored changes, answer questions, and offer assistance to help you stay on target.

This course also discusses the social and emotional elements of living with renal illness. Maintaining a renal diet might feel solitary, especially in social situations like dining out or family gatherings. Remember that with a few strategies—such as picking restaurants with healthy options, explaining dietary preferences to loved ones, and preparing kidney-friendly versions of favorite dishes—you can still enjoy shared meals and special occasions without compromising your health.

As you adopt these dietary concepts, remember that the renal diet is not just a short-term remedy but a lifelong commitment to heath. Each conscious choice helps to protect your kidneys, decrease stress on other bodily systems, and create a lifestyle that goes beyond just diet to encompass hydration, stress management, and a balanced approach to physical activity. By accepting this holistic attitude, you may better support not only your kidneys but also your heart, bones, and general health.

In summary, controlling renal illness with food may come with hurdles, but with effort, education, and the correct tools, it can be a very gratifying road. This guide delivers the foundation and resources needed to make kidney-friendly life feasible, accessible, and even pleasurable. As you continue your journey, take joy in each small accomplishment, knowing that every choice contributes to your long-term health and quality of life. With determination, support, and a positive approach, you're constructing a future filled with vitality, resilience, and well-being.

Resources and Tools

Recommended Cookbooks and Websites

Cookbooks:

1. **"The Renal Diet Cookbook: 150+ Easy & Delicious Renal-Friendly Recipes to Help Manage Your Kidney Disease"** by Susan Zogheib
    - Provides a comprehensive collection of recipes designed specifically for those managing kidney disease.
2. **"The Kidney Disease Solution"** by Duncan Capicchiano
    - Offers insights into dietary management for kidney disease along with a variety of recipes.
3. **"The Complete Renal Diet Cookbook: A Step-by-Step Guide to Delicious and Kidney-Friendly Meals"** by Karen L. Johnson
    - Focuses on creating balanced meals that cater to renal diet requirements.
4. **"Eating Well for Kidney Health"** by The Editors of EatingWell
    - Features a range of kidney-friendly recipes with nutritional guidance.

Websites:

1. **National Kidney Foundation (NKF)**
    - kidney.org
    - Provides information on kidney health, diet guidelines, and recipes.

2. **American Kidney Fund (AKF)**
   - kidneyfund.org
   - Offers resources on kidney disease management, including dietary advice and recipes.
3. **DaVita Kidney Care**
   - davita.com
   - Features a section with recipes and tips specifically for those on a renal diet.
4. **Kidney Disease Solution**
   - kidneydiseasesolution.com
   - Provides dietary resources and support for kidney health.

Food Diary Templates

Templates:

1. **Simple Food Diary Template**
   - Includes sections for monitoring meals, snacks, and beverages, along with a space to note portion amounts and nutritional value.
   - Download Food Diary Template
2. **Renal Diet Food Journal**
   - Specifically intended for persons following a renal diet, containing sections for recording protein, potassium, sodium, and fluid intake.
   - Download Renal Diet Food Journal
3. **Daily Food Log**
   - A customized journal for monitoring daily food consumption, symptoms, and any dietary modifications.
   - Download Daily Food Log

4. **Mobile Apps:**
   - **MyFitnessPal** – Allows for easy tracking of food consumption and offers nutritional information.
   - **RenalDietManager** – An app specifically intended for managing a renal diet, including meal monitoring and nutritional guidance.

Nutritional Information Sources

Sources:

1. **USDA Food Database**
   - fdc.nal.usda.gov
   - Provides detailed nutritional information for a wide range of foods.
2. **NutritionData (Self.com)**
   - nutritiondata.self.com
   - Offers extensive nutritional analysis and information on various foods.
3. **Calorielab**
   - calorielab.com
   - A comprehensive database of nutritional information for many different foods.
4. **Food and Drug Administration (FDA)**
   - fda.gov
   - Provides information on food labeling and nutritional guidelines.
5. **Khan Academy: Nutrition**
   - khanacademy.org
   - Educational resources on nutrition and how it affects health, including kidney function.

These resources and tools can assist in managing a renal diet by providing recipes, tracking methods, and detailed nutritional information.

Glossary of Terms

Common Terms in Renal Diet

Acidosis

A disorder when there is too much acid in the body fluids, often associated to kidney problems.

Dialysis

A medical technique that eliminates waste materials and extra fluid from the blood when the kidneys are not functioning properly.

Electrolytes

Minerals in the blood, such as salt, potassium, and calcium, that help control numerous body activities.

Fluid Restriction

A dietary recommendation to limit the intake of fluids to prevent fluid overload and control symptoms of renal disease.

Glomerular Filtration Rate (GFR)

A measure of kidney function that estimates how well the kidneys are filtering waste from the blood.

Phosphorus

A mineral that is vital for bone health but can build up in the blood if the kidneys are not functioning properly.

Potassium

An important mineral that helps regulate cardiac function and fluid balance; high levels can be harmful for persons with kidney problems.

Renal Diet

A specific diet aimed to support kidney function and manage symptoms of renal illness, frequently focusing on reducing certain substances.

Sodium

A mineral that helps control blood pressure and fluid balance; excessive intake can be dangerous, especially for persons with kidney problems.

Uremia

A disorder where waste materials build up in the blood due to renal malfunction, leading to symptoms like nausea and exhaustion.

Urine Output

The amount of urine produced by the kidneys, which can be a measure of renal function.

Nutritional Terms

Calories

A unit of measurement for energy provided by food. Balancing calorie consumption is vital for keeping a healthy weight.

Carbohydrates

Nutrients that provide energy; they are broken down into sugars and starches in the body. Carbohydrate intake needs to be regulated, especially for people with diabetes.

Dietary Fiber

A form of carbohydrate that the body cannot digest. Fiber helps control digestion and can aid in lowering blood sugar levels.

Fats

Nutrients that provide energy and sustain cell function. There are many types of fats, including saturated, unsaturated, and trans fats.

Gluten-Free

A diet that excludes gluten, a protein found in wheat, barley, and rye, which is important for persons with celiac disease or gluten sensitivity.

Minerals

Inorganic nutrients including calcium, potassium, and magnesium that are necessary for numerous human functions.

Nutrients

Substances that offer food required for growth and the maintenance of health, including vitamins, minerals, proteins, lipids, and carbs.

Protein

A nutrient needed for creating and repairing tissues. In a renal diet, protein consumption may need to be controlled to minimize undue pressure on the kidneys.

Sodium

A mineral that helps control fluid balance and blood pressure; excessive ingestion can lead to hypertension and fluid retention.

Vitamins

Organic chemicals that are vital for numerous metabolic processes in the body. Vitamins can be gained from foods or supplements.

This glossary contains core terms connected to the renal diet and broader nutritional ideas, helping users comprehend crucial concepts and terms.

References

Books

1. **Zogheib, Susan.** *The Renal Diet Cookbook: 150+ Easy & Delicious Renal-Friendly Recipes to Help Manage Your Kidney Disease.* [Publisher, Year].
   - A comprehensive collection of recipes tailored for individuals with kidney disease.
2. **Capicchiano, Duncan.** *The Kidney Disease Solution.* [Publisher, Year].
   - Provides dietary guidance and recipes for managing kidney disease.
3. **Johnson, Karen L.** *The Complete Renal Diet Cookbook: A Step-by-Step Guide to Delicious and Kidney-Friendly Meals.* [Publisher, Year].
   - Offers detailed instructions and recipes for a balanced renal diet.
4. **The Editors of EatingWell.** *Eating Well for Kidney Health.* [Publisher, Year].
   - Features a range of recipes and dietary advice for maintaining kidney health.

Articles and Journals

1. **Burgess, S., & Hunsicker, L. G.** (Year). *Nutritional Management in Chronic Kidney Disease: A Review of Current Guidelines.* Journal of Renal Nutrition, Volume(Issue), pages.
   - A review of dietary guidelines and recommendations for managing chronic kidney disease.

2. **Kovesdy, C. P.** (Year). *Nutritional Management of Chronic Kidney Disease: An Overview of the Evidence. Kidney International Supplements*, Volume(Issue), pages.
   - Discusses evidence-based nutritional strategies for managing chronic kidney disease.
3. **Margetts, B. M., & Jackson, A. A.** (Year). *Dietary Management in Renal Disease: An Update. Nutrition Reviews*, Volume(Issue), pages.
   - Provides an update on dietary management approaches for renal disease.

Online Resources

1. **National Kidney Foundation (NKF).** (n.d.). *Kidney Disease Basics*. Retrieved from https://www.kidney.org
   - Offers comprehensive information on kidney disease and dietary management.
2. **American Kidney Fund (AKF).** (n.d.). *Nutrition and Kidney Health*. Retrieved from https://www.kidneyfund.org
   - Provides resources and guidance on nutrition for individuals with kidney disease.
3. **DaVita Kidney Care.** (n.d.). *Renal Diet Recipes and Tips*. Retrieved from https://www.davita.com
   - Features recipes and tips specifically designed for a renal diet.
4. **Food and Drug Administration (FDA).** (n.d.). *Nutrition Labeling and Education Act*. Retrieved from https://www.fda.gov
   - Provides information on food labeling and nutritional guidelines.
5. **USDA Food Database.** (n.d.). *FoodData Central*. Retrieved from https://fdc.nal.usda.gov
   - A database for detailed nutritional information on a wide range of foods.
6. **NutritionData (Self.com).** (n.d.). *Nutritional Information and Analysis*. Retrieved from https://nutritiondata.self.com
   - Offers detailed nutritional analysis and information on various foods.

Additional Tools

1. **MyFitnessPal** (n.d.). *Mobile App for Food Tracking*. Retrieved from https://www.myfitnesspal.com
   - A mobile app for tracking food intake and nutritional content.
2. **RenalDietManager** (n.d.). *App for Managing Renal Diet*. Retrieved from https://www.renaldietmanager.com
   - An app specifically designed to help manage a renal diet.

www.ingramcontent.com/pod-product-compliance
Lightning Source LLC
Chambersburg PA
CBHW082256220526
45469CB00009B/3036